HEALTHY!

BEAUTIFUL INSIDE AND OUT

SHARI WARE, Founder of FAB New Body

Book a complimentary 30-minute call with me to find your healthy!

https://calendly.com/shari-ware/30min

Connect with me on Facebook: https://www.facebook.com/shariwarefab

Connect with me on my Facebook Page: https://www.facebook.com/fabnewbody

Connect with me on Instagram: https://www.instagram.com/shariwarefab

Connect with me on Twitter: https://twitter.com/shariwarefab

Connect with me on Linked In: https://www.linkedin.com/in/shariware

1 Best Selling Author of Fat to Fabulous – Diet Free Weight Loss for Real Women

You can get the book here: https://amzn.to/2E0sqSI

FEATURED IN...

DISCLAIMER

The people and events described and depicted in this book are for educational purposes only. While every attempt has been made to verify information provided in this book, the author assumes no responsibility for any errors, inaccuracies or omissions.

If advice concerning medical matters is needed, the services of a qualified professional should be sought. This book is not intended for use as a source of medical advice.

The examples within this book are not intended to represent or guarantee that everyone or anyone will achieve their desired results. Each individual's success will be determined by his or her desire, dedication, effort and motivation. There are no guarantees you will achieve your desired outcome; the tools, stories and information are provided as examples only.

First Edition 2018 | Copyright 2018 by Shari Ware

Table of Contents

Introduction

Do you have a weight problem? Do you look in the mirror every day and hate what you see? Do you avoid looking in the mirror because you don't like what you know will be reflected? Do you secretly envy skinny, bikini-clad women and wish desperately you could be like them?

I used to say *yes* to all of the above!

I started putting on weight from around the age of five and by the time I was 33, I was at my heaviest at over 180kg. Long story short (you can read my first book, Fat to Fabulous - Diet Free Weight Loss for Real Women for the long story - it can be found at https://amzn.to/2E0sqSI), I lost 100kg by changing my lifestyle, starting with my nutrition.

I learned so much over my 100kg weight release journey but the learning didn't stop there. I have learned so much MORE since. The biggest thing I've learned is that I knew absolutely nothing about nutrition and so many other things that have a massive impact on our HEALTH. Yes, I lost 100kg, but I did it in a way that I wouldn't recommend to anyone and in a way that was definitely not sustainable. There are much healthier ways to release weight than the vehicle I used, which was sticking to 1200 calories per day.

Back then, I simply didn't know any better and I know that you, just like me, don't know what you don't know. Which is why I decided to write this book. I want to help you to understand what is important and why. I want to clear up some things that might be confusing you and making you wonder which is the best option for you.

There are so many weight loss gurus and programs on the market and many of them tell you conflicting information. Who is telling the truth? Who should you listen to? How do you know what will work for you?

Have you asked yourself these questions? I know I did and I still do!

Why Read This Book?

The aim of this book is to help clear up some common misconceptions. It will help you understand more about your emotional eating and why it isn't your fault. It will help you understand how your lack of self-love plays a role and you'll learn ways to improve it.

I address the fact that transformation starts on the inside and that the physical changes will follow and teach you about healthy choices that make a massive impact on your health. Lastly, but certainly not least, we'll talk about the fact that YOU are important.

If you are ready to find YOUR healthy, then dive right in! You'll find this book is not very long. I've kept it short and sweet because I wanted to give you the information you need in the shortest possible time so you can spend more time IMPLEMENTING!

They say that knowledge is power but that's not exactly true. Knowledge is only power if you *implement* what you learn. My hope is this book will help you do that. With this aim in mind, I give you an easy, healthy change you can make at the end of each chapter so you can start improving your health from the very first day.

Always remember you CAN change your story, one change at a time!

Let's Work Together!

PS – if you need some help with changing your story to a much better one, please reach out to me and book in for your free 30-minute call to get you started on your journey. I can help you to get clarity about what your next step should be. You don't need to know ALL the steps, just the next one. You'll find that when you take that first step, the next one will be presented to you and the next one and the next. So, take that first step today and book your call at https://calendly.com/shari-ware/30min

You CAN change your story, ONE change at a time.

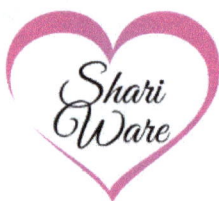

Shari Ware

Chapter One

HEALTHY!

Healthy. What does it mean? Well, first let me tell you a few things it DOESN'T mean:

- Healthy DOESN'T mean skinny
- Healthy DOESN'T mean fit

Now I'm not saying skinny or fit people aren't healthy and I'm not saying they are. What I am saying is that just because a person is skinny, doesn't mean they are necessarily healthy and the same for a fit person.

For instance, there are people out there who have genetics that mean they can pretty much eat whatever they want and don't get fat. Some of them eat healthily and some of them don't eat very healthily at all. Some of them think that because they don't gain weight it doesn't matter what they eat. What they don't realise is that whilst they may not have health problems in the short term, over the long term they will. And we are seeing this happening so much in today's society.

The same goes for 'fit' people. Just because someone is fit, doesn't necessarily mean they are healthy. There are several factors that go into being the healthiest we can be and exercise is only one of them. Have you ever heard of someone in the prime of their life who seems perfectly fit and healthy suddenly dying from a heart attack? Exercise is an important factor in creating a healthy body but it can be taken to extremes just like anything else and when it is, it is NOT healthy.

So, I have spoken about a couple of misconceptions that many people have about the word 'healthy' but there are a couple more I want to address before we go any further:

- Fat people are lazy
- It's as easy as watching what you eat and exercising
- It doesn't matter WHAT you eat as long as you have a calorie deficit – it's all about calories in vs calories out

Ever heard of these ones? Ever been at the receiving end of one or more of these or maybe even all of them? I have and for many years I believed them, even during most of my 100kg weight release journey. I just didn't know any better. I didn't know what I didn't know and I absolutely know there are so many others out there like me.

If you believe these misconceptions or "myths", then YOU are one of those people and I am so glad you're reading this book!

I want you to know you are NOT lazy. Louise Hay said it best:

"Weight is just a physical manifestation of a much deeper issue."

We will talk about some of those in later chapters.

I want you to know it's NOT as easy as watching what you eat and exercising. I want you to know that it absolutely DOES matter what you eat and that it is NOT all about calories in vs calories out! If you decided all you wanted to eat is doughnuts and so you ate 1200 calories worth of doughnuts every day, would you have a calorie deficit? Yes, you would. Would you be healthy? NO, you would NOT. Of course it matters what you eat and we will also address this in a later chapter.

I also want you to know it's NOT your fault! There is definitely a way to find YOUR healthy and it CAN be so much easier than you believe it is going to be. If you do have weight to lose, I want you to know that *healthy* is way more important than *skinny* and by concentrating on making healthier choices, the weight will fall away anyway.

FIND YOUR HEALTHY ACTION STEP

1. List two healthy changes you know you could make:

   _____

   _____

2. Pick one and start making the change today!

3. Watch my video at https://youtu.be/Z8TVmy51Oyc to learn how to successfully implement your changes.

It is health
that is real
wealth,
not pieces of
gold and
silver

- Mahatma Gandhi

Chapter Two

EMOTIONAL EATING

Emotional eating is when we're triggered to eat 'off plan'. When we're on a journey to better health, we usually have an eating plan of some kind we try to stick to. Sometimes we choose to have an 'off plan' meal or day which is completely ok and totally necessary for some of us if we're going to stick to our healthy eating regime for the rest of our lives – which is what we're aiming to do.

So why is emotional eating a problem? It becomes a problem when it makes you lose control of your eating because there are so many repercussions both mentally and physically. When you give in to emotional eating, it usually makes you feel angry and guilty at the very least.

It can actually cause a whole lot of negative emotions and quite often makes people think about giving up on their healthy eating plan. Also, if you're trying to reach a health goal it can seriously set you back.

There are 5 main triggers that cause us to emotionally eat:

- Eating to silence emotions
- Loneliness or boredom
- Habits from childhood
- Social Occasions
- Chronic Stress

Eating to Silence Emotions

Eating to silence our emotions is when something happens that makes us feel either angry or sad and we just want to eat some chocolate or a piece of cheesecake or maybe even open a bottle of wine. We feel bad and we try to make ourselves feel better by eating and or drinking some kind of comfort food.

Loneliness or Boredom

Then there is the loneliness or boredom trigger. How many times have you found yourself sitting on the couch watching TV and sticking your hand in a bag of chips until they're all gone? Or eating half a block of chocolate or a packet of tim tams without even realising?

Habits from Childhood

Habits from our childhood is a sneaky one. I know this happened to me when I was a child and I even did the same with my own children. Good behaviour calls for a treat, right? You did well at school and got a great report card so your parents took you out for pizza or ice-cream or sometimes even both? Treating ourselves with food can be a hard habit to break!

Social Occasions

So many family and social occasions revolve around food. Birthdays, Christmas, Easter, weddings... the list is endless. When we get together on these occasions, it's very easy to lose control.

Chronic Stress

Last but certainly not least, chronic stress is one of the most common of the emotional eating triggers and in this modern-day world, it is literally all around us. Financial stress, stress at work, emotional stress, lack of sleep. It can cause us to make some really bad food choices and there is a scientific reason for that.

When we're under stress, our body goes into 'fight or flight' or 'survival' mode. Our bodies can't distinguish between the stress of lack of sleep as opposed to the stress of being chased by a tiger. To our brain, it is exactly the same thing and causes the same response in our body.

A couple of things happen when our body goes into this mode. Firstly, the body will want to replenish the calories it feels it has used after needing to either fight or run away from the danger and so it makes you want to eat. It also raises the amount of cortisol in your body which makes you hungry for sugary, fatty foods.

What kinds of foods do you go looking for when you're stressed? I'm pretty sure it isn't a piece of fruit or a salad!

Another thing that happens when the body is under stress is it shuts down any function it doesn't need to survive. Fat burning is one of those functions. Your body will actually start to store fat in case it needs it to fight or run away again. Our bodies are very, *very* smart and they only do what they need to do to keep us safe. Sometimes we think our bodies are working against us, but I absolutely promise you that's NOT the case.

14

Emotional eating can seriously undo all your hard work if you aren't careful and learn how to control it. Control it you say? How can you do that? It is possible and I have a technique that I'll share with you later. It will help you control your emotional eating in as little as five minutes. It has helped so many of my clients to overcome their emotional eating and it can help you too!

One of my beautiful clients had this to say:

"I had read Fat to Fabulous: Diet Free Weight Loss for Real Women, by Shari Ware, and loved her weight release journey. She is real, human and had faced her own weight issues. I was interested in Shari's ongoing journey so I started following her on Facebook. Then, I participated in her Emotional Eating Audits, and the 30 Day YEESS! Program. I also had a one-on-one consultation with Shari to discuss my emotional eating issues. Attending Shari's weight release programs has made a huge impact on my life.

I have now applied the fat to fabulous steps into my weight release journey. I find Shari's programs motivating and she gives you practical steps and life changes that you can easily incorporate into your busy lifestyle.

In conjunction with another weight loss program and Shari's weight release support and guidance, I have lost 31kgs.

Shari has helped me change my emotional eating issues and has given me invaluable advice to use when I feel tempted to emotional eat. With the lifetime skills I have gained, I am able to work through, and overcome my emotional eating triggers. I am on my way to a happy and healthy version of myself. Shari Ware has changed my life! I cannot thank, or praise her enough for helping me gain my life back." - Catherine

FIND YOUR HEALTHY ACTION STEP

1. Use the checklist on the next page to determine your two most common triggers and write them here:

    _____

    _____

2. Watch my video at https://youtu.be/2U0MwcK6NNY to learn my golden technique to help you control your emotional eating in as little as five minutes!

3. Use this technique when you're triggered to eat off plan.

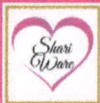

Discover Your Emotional Eating Triggers

CHECKLIST

FAB
NEW BODY

A) DO YOU EAT WHEN....

- [ ] You're angry?
- [ ] You want to feel happy?
- [ ] You do feel happy?
- [ ] You're sad?

B) DO YOU EAT WHEN....

- [ ] You're bored?
- [ ] You're watching tv?
- [ ] You're procrastinating?
- [ ] You're lonely?

C) DO YOU EAT WHEN....

- [ ] You've had a win?
- [ ] You've achieved a goal?
- [ ] You're disappointed?
- [ ] You're celebrating?

D) DO YOU EAT MORE WHEN...

- [ ] You're at a party?
- [ ] Someone offers you food?
- [ ] It's a special holiday?
- [ ] You're at a family feast?

E) DO YOU EAT WHEN....

- [ ] You're tired?
- [ ] You're stressed?
- [ ] You're under pressure?
- [ ] You're avoiding problems?

THE 5 MOST COMMON TRIGGERS

A) Eating to silence emotions
B) Loneliness or boredom
C) Habits from childhood
D) Social occasions
E) Chronic stress

If you have 2 or more ticks in a section, it is one of your emotional eating triggers

No amount of icecream has ever been able to mend a broken heart

= Laura Houssain

Chapter Three

ATTITUDE

A is for ATTITUDE! Are you a glass half empty or a glass half full kind of person? This may not seem like it matters and if you're talking about how full a glass is, it probably doesn't, but the point I'm making is that your ATTITUDE can either help or hinder your progress to creating a healthier life.

We tell ourselves stories all the time, sometimes without realising it. But the story we tell ourselves may make it harder for us to achieve our goals. For instance, say you're trying to make healthier food choices which means you're choosing not to eat certain things. There are two ways of looking at it:

Some people choose the story of, *"I have to give up those foods or I won't lose weight."*

What's wrong with that I hear you ask? Well, what if instead of telling ourselves THAT story, we told ourselves the story, *"I am choosing to make healthier food choices because I know it will make me feel amazing!"*

You tell me which is the better story and which one will help you achieve your goal?

Lack

So often we have an attitude of *lack*. We tell ourselves we have to give things up to achieve our goals. Does that make you feel

21

better or worse? Does that make achieving your goal easier or harder?

No one made you set that goal for yourself. No one is making you do anything. So instead of approaching it with an attitude of lack or having to sacrifice, have the attitude that you are *choosing* to make healthy food choices and put a whole new perspective on it.

I Can't

Another story we tell ourselves is the 'I can't' story. Here are examples of the classics:

- I can't lose weight because...
- I can't exercise because...

There are many, *many* more but ain't nobody got time for that!

Instead of telling yourself you can't, what would happen if you told yourself you could? I'll tell you what would happen. You WOULD! How do I know? Because if I had told myself I couldn't lose 100kg, then I wouldn't have. If I had told myself I couldn't run a marathon, then I wouldn't have. I was able to achieve both of those things because I told myself I COULD and I DID despite the challenges along the way, of which there were many!

You CAN do ANYTHING you tell yourself you can!

Your Past

Where else can attitude make a difference? Your attitude toward your past. Without realising it, many of us let negative things that happened in our past impact negatively on our lives.

Your past is NOT how your story ends. Your story ends however you want it to end. Your story ends the way you *make* it end by what you do every day from now until the day you die. So if you have been letting your past hold you back, now is the time to change that and change that you can.

The Blame Game

There may be a reason why your health is not where it should be that's not your fault. We are now seeing so many health issues that have come about due to a lifetime of poor nutrition and exercise.

In some cases, it may not be your fault. In some cases, it absolutely is NOT your fault. However, just because it isn't your fault doesn't mean it's not your responsibility. Does it matter whose fault it is in the end? What really matters? Getting healthy is what really matters. So no matter how you got to this point in your life, just know that the only person who can change it is YOU!

Regardless of who is to blame, it's YOUR responsibility and only yours to change it.

Perfectionism

Have you ever tried to make a change but gave up because it wasn't executed perfectly? How about when you're on a 'diet', eat something off plan and then keep eating off plan because you've already 'ruined the diet'?

I like to use the analogy of dropping your phone for this one. If you drop your phone, do you say, *"Oh well, I already dropped it so I will just keep jumping on it and break it some more"*? No! Of course you don't! That doesn't make any sense at all.

Neither does the 'already ruined my diet so I will just keep going' story.

The point I'm trying to make is having a perfectionist attitude won't help you. It's ok for things not to be perfect. Imperfect change is ALWAYS better than NO change!

FIND YOUR HEALTHY ACTION STEP

1. List two negative attitudes you want to change:

    _____

    _____

2. Get a red pen and cross them out!

3. Write two new POSITIVE attitudes below in your favourite colour!

    _____

    _____

A healthy attitude is contagious but don't wait to catch it from somone else. Be a carrier.

= Tom Stoppard

Chapter Four

LOVE YOURSELF

Love yourself. A whole chapter about loving yourself. Why? Because it's frickin' important, that's why!

Have you ever heard of a thing called self-sabotage? You know, when you're trying really hard to make changes and you're doing really well and you seem like you're on a roll... and then something happens... and you get derailed and it's all over red rover?

It's not a question of IF this has happened to you. The question is HOW MANY TIMES has it happened?!

So why do we self-sabotage? There are a few reasons and one of them definitely comes back to how much we love ourselves.

Here are some of the beliefs many struggling with their weight and their health have. Sometimes they're not even aware of them:

- I am not enough
- I am not worthy
- I am not lovable
- I am not important

How did it make you feel when you read those statements? Did they strike a chord? I would bet money they did!

When you get to a point that you feel you're doing really well, these beliefs rear their ugly head from deep in your subconscious and you self-sabotage to prove the beliefs are true.

Sound ridiculous, right? I totally agree! It is utterly ridiculous, but that's how powerful the subconscious mind is. So strap yourself in because boy, do we have some work to do!

Ask yourself this question... "Do I REALLY love myself?"

Here is another one for ya... "Do I love myself UNCONDITIONALLY?"

And a few more...

- Am I deserving?
- Am I worthy?
- Am I important?

And the clincher... "Am I ENOUGH?"

If you didn't answer all those questions with a resounding "HELL YEAH!" then you best get working on that self-love thing I'm talkin' about.

What happens when you can say "HELL YEAH!" to all of those questions? It means whenever you set yourself a goal you REALLY want to achieve, you won't have to worry about that sneaky little self-sabotage demon sneaking in telling you you're not good enough or not deserving enough to achieve it.

The most awesome part is you don't even have to get all the way there before you start to achieve your goals. Just being *aware* of these beliefs and consciously working on eliminating them helps to get the subconscious mind onboard. Then, it will be even easier to achieve your health goals or any other goals you set for yourself.

Not loving myself was one of the main reasons why I was unsuccessful at releasing weight for so many years. I didn't like what I saw in the mirror every day. I didn't love that person staring back at me. That person wasn't important, wasn't worthy, wasn't deserving and wasn't enough. I tried so many times to release the weight and at times, I would have success. I would be on that 'roll' that we get on and then those subconscious beliefs would start creeping in slowly. I would self-sabotage and be right back at square one if not even further back from where I had started. I'm sure you know exactly what I'm talking about because you've been there too.

Once I became conscious of those beliefs buried deep in my psyche, I started to slowly work on them and I continue to work on them to this day.

I can already hear you asking, *"How do I know if I have subconscious beliefs that are holding me back?"* I will be honest with you. It can be tricky at times. The subconscious mind always has your best interests at heart and always wants to protect you. Sometimes that means that it deliberately hides things from you because it doesn't think that you can handle it.

That doesn't mean you should give up though. The only way you are going to uncover those beliefs is to consciously work on uncovering them. By doing so, you're telling your subconscious mind you're ready and at the perfect time, whatever you need to know WILL be revealed to you.

The first place to start is to get a blank journal you can write in. Take some time out alone and ask yourself the question, *"What do I believe about myself to be true?"* and then just write. Keep asking yourself the question and write whatever comes into your mind. You might be amazed at some of the things you uncover!

It's amazing to see the changes we can make in our lives when we love ourselves. I see the changes in my beautiful clients every day. I realised not so long ago that I don't really help people to release weight – I help them to love themselves and when they love themselves, they make healthier choices and the weight release follows. It makes my heart sing!

If you would like to be one of my gorgeous clients who I help to love unconditionally what they see in the mirror every single day with the extra support of one-on-one mentoring, book in for your first complimentary session at https://calendly.com/shari-ware/30min

So, what can you do now to love yourself more? There are so many different things and as I always say, different strokes for different folks. I will give you a list of things you can try out and see if they work for you at the end of this chapter, but first, let me tell you what my daily self-love ritual is.

The first thing I do when I get out of bed in the morning – after I go pee of course! – is to do something that Louise Hay did. Every morning Louise Hay would go to the mirror, look herself in the eye and tell herself how much she loved herself. When I first heard that I decided I would start to do it too.

I have to say, the first time I tried it I couldn't look myself in the eye and say it. I was amazed at just how much I DIDN'T love myself! I still said the words though and I continued to do it every morning and each morning it got a little easier. Now, I can totally look myself in the eye in that mirror and say to myself, *"Shari Ware, I really, really love you! You are amazing!"* I actually throw in a few choice words as well, but they are not fit to be printed in a book!

I usually do it naked (TMI!) and I look at my body with all my lumps and bumps and tell my legs how much I love them because they have gotten me through so many years of having to lug around 180kg. I tell my body that I love it so much for not failing on me when I really needed it and that I love it because it is so strong! After I've told myself how much I love ME, I recite a poem written by a lovely colleague of mine, Lois Lovegrove, which you can see on the next page.

♥

MY PROMISE

I LOVE EVERY PART OF MYSELF AND I COMPLETELY EMBRACE ALL OF MYSELF.

I HONOUR ALL OF THE GIFTS I HAVE BEEN GIVEN AND ALL OF THE KNOWLEDGE I HAVE GAINED.

I RESPECT MYSELF AND ALL THAT I HAVE OVERCOME TO BE THE PERSON I AM TODAY.

I FORGIVE MYSELF FOR ALL OF THE CHOICES THAT I HAVE MADE THAT HAVEN'T SERVED ME TO MY HIGHEST AND BEST.

I PROMISE THAT I WILL ALWAYS LOVE, HONOUR AND RESPECT MYSELF AND THAT I WILL LIVE MY LIFE TO MY HIGHEST POTENTIAL.

ME

LOISLOVEGROVE.COM

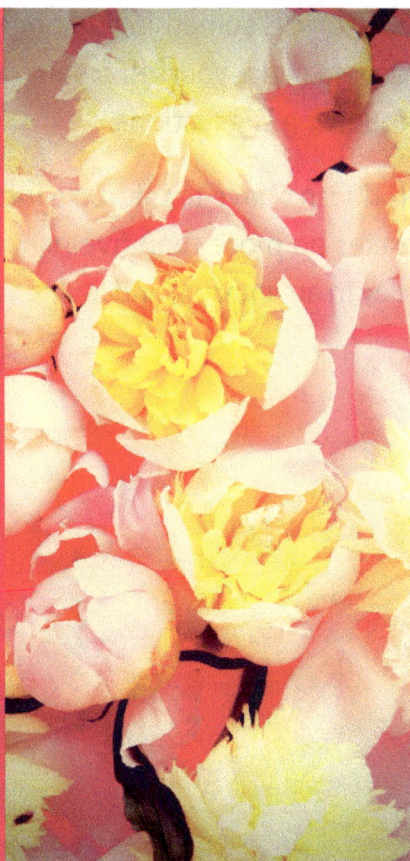

Self-love is something that needs to be worked on every single day, so make yourself a daily self-love ritual using some of the following suggestions.

It doesn't have to take up a lot of time. My daily self-love ritual takes no more than five minutes, but it helps me to start my day in an amazing and loving way.

10 WAYS YOU CAN PRACTICE SELF LOVE

1. Marry yourself – actually have a ceremony where you marry yourself. Why? Because you are going to be with YOU for the REST of your life! There is an awesome TED talk on this subject which I highly recommend. I even made my daughter watch it. You can check it out at https://youtu.be/P3fIZuW9P_M

2. Massage lotion or oil into your body and as you massage each part, tell it how much you love that particular body part for being with you through all of life's ups and downs.

3. Listen to self-love meditations, podcasts, audiobooks, etc.

4. Buy YOURSELF flowers.

5. Nourish your body with healthy food – you can CHOOSE to eat healthy because you love yourself!

6. Take a bath with beautiful bath salts or oils.

7. Write in a gratitude journal – I do this every day. Firstly, I write down the names of at least three people I want to send love or healing to. Then I write a list of ten things I'm grateful for. The first four things on the list are the same every day: my beautiful daughter Nataasjia, my

amazing life, my wonderful health, and my awesome fitness. And finally, I write down six different things I'm grateful for that day.

8. Buy yourself a beautiful piece of jewellery to symbolise your love for yourself.

9. Create a self-love calendar.

10. Create a separate fund for self-love practices and experiences.

FIND YOUR HEALTHY ACTION STEP

1. Create your own self-love ritual below!

_____

_____

_____

_____

Love yourself first and everything else falls in line.

— Lucille Ball

CHAPTER 5

TRANSFORMATION STARTS ON THE INSIDE

If you want to transform your life in any way, whether it be your health, your body, your finances, your relationships or your career, it's not as simple as setting a goal and *voila!* it all comes together.

What most people don't realise is that transformation starts on the inside.

Yes, you can set a goal, decide what you need to do to attain that goal and then implement the steps you need to implement. Sometimes we do all those things and we succeed... and sometimes we don't!

So, what's the real difference between success and failure? Your heart and your subconscious mind are not on board. That's the difference. If you truly want to transform and have that transformation be long-lasting, your head and your heart have to be in it.

Firstly, you have to have a massive WHY. It has to be so big that it strikes you right to the core every time you think about it. Why does it have to be so big? Because for every why that we have, there are usually just as many why nots, if not more!

Our why nots are those reasons why we DON'T want to make the changes we know we need to make. Here are some why nots you might have come across:

- I can't afford to eat healthily
- I don't have time to exercise
- I don't want to give up my junk food

Have you experienced any of these before? How many times have you started working towards transforming a part of your life only to give up because it all seemed too hard? That's because your head and your heart weren't in it to begin with. That's because what I call your WHY Power wasn't strong enough to overcome all the why nots you had.

When you have massive WHY Power, you don't NEED willpower! You'll do whatever you need to do to achieve your transformation. It doesn't mean the journey will be a perfect one, but you WILL cross the finish line in the end.

So, how do you find your massive WHY Power? Make it EMOTIONAL! It absolutely has to strike you right in the heart when you think about it. This is where the HEART comes into it.

Let me give you an example. When I was at my biggest, I was over 180kg and I knew that at that weight, it was only a matter of time before I had some serious health issues. I lived in fear of having a major heart attack and dying AND I was a single parent of a young daughter.

You would think that alone was a massive WHY and it was. But not massive enough. It wasn't enough because unfortunately, I had a massive why not – I didn't want to have another relationship. I'd had a bad relationship experience where I had been hurt very badly and I didn't want to repeat that. Which is why I was so overweight in the first place. It was my suit of armour. It was my way of making myself so unattractive that I wouldn't be appealing to the opposite sex and it worked extremely well!

One morning I woke up and realised that one day my beautiful girl was going to be moving out, as is the natural order of things. I realised that when that eventually did happen, IF I was still alive, I was going to be at home, sitting on the couch, ALONE. It was in that instant that I realised I no longer wanted to be alone. I was open to the possibility of a relationship and, in fact, I decided that it was definitely something I wanted.

At that point, my WHY Power was doubly powerful because my massive why not had flipped into a why! My massive why became wanting to see my daughter finish high school, go to university, get married and have children AND to find a partner to LIVE my life with.

Do you understand why your WHY Power is so important?

Now, while your WHY Power is super important, something else is essential when it comes to creating transformation in your life – BELIEF. And belief has three important pillars.

First, we need to believe that what we want to achieve is *possible* in the first place. If we don't believe that it IS possible, why would we even TRY to achieve it? We wouldn't. It's as simple as that.

The second part is you have to believe in *yourself*. You have to believe that *you* can achieve that goal you have set for yourself.

The third part is one I have only just recently realised and that is the importance of what you believe *about yourself*. The beliefs about yourself that go right to your very core and that you live your life by, whether you are aware of them or not. We talked about some of those in the previous chapter. You remember, that whole chapter about self-love and how frickin' important it is?

The extremely interesting thing about our beliefs about ourselves is that quite often, for transformation to occur they have to change. How do I know this? Well, as I said before, this is something I have only just come to realise very recently and I came to that realisation when I was doing a business exercise.

I was having to describe my 'Ideal Customer Avatar'. Basically, the ideal person that I'm trying to help. We had to choose a particular person who was our ideal customer and answer a great big long list of questions about them to get to know them better.

For me, those kinds of exercises are always a bit easier because *I am* my ideal customer avatar. When I say *I am*, I mean the person I was back when I was 180kg. When answering the questions, I had to think back to what the answer would have been back when I was *that* person.

There was one question in particular that gave me one of the most massive 'a-ha!' moments of my life and I can tell you I have had a few of those moments so far!

The question was, *"What are her life beliefs?"*

It seems like such a simple question. I thought back to the person I was then and I started to write. I wrote three things:

1. Everything happens for a reason (I still believe this!)

2. Others are more important

3. I'm a bad person

When I wrote those down and sat back and really looked at what I had written, I realised that I subconsciously had those beliefs back then and that totally blew me away. I realised those last two beliefs had absolutely changed and that if they HADN'T changed, I would still be over 180kg today.

So you see, true, long-lasting transformation starts from the inside. It starts from inside your head and from inside your heart. If you want to truly transform your life, start going within rather than looking for answers outside of yourself.

FIND YOUR HEALTHY ACTION STEP

1. List your massive WHY and your biggest WHY NOT below:

    _____

    _____

2. Is your WHY massive enough to overcome your WHY NOT? If not, what can you work on to change that?

    _____

    _____

3. List two core life beliefs that you have about yourself:

    _____

    _____

4. Write down any beliefs you need to change:

    _____

    _____

You must find the place inside yourself where nothing is impossible

- Deepak Chopra

Chapter Six

HEALTHIER CHOICES

This chapter is all about healthier choices you can make that will positively impact on your health. Remember, it's not about being perfect. I've learned that being healthy is more about balance.

You don't have to give up all the things you love. Maybe there are some things you know you could benefit from reducing, but that's something only you can know and change. In the meantime, here are ten things you can do that will immediately improve your health, even if you only pick one to start working on.

DRINK WATER!

I'm putting this first because it's the easiest one. I mean, really, how hard is it to drink more water if you really try?

Did you know that the minute you feel thirsty, you're already dehydrated? Dehydration slows down your metabolism, so if you ARE trying to release weight, you need to get your water intake right.

There are other important reasons for you to you drink enough water, including flushing toxins from your body and helping the kidneys excrete waste through urination. Water also boosts the production of cells and when your body is hydrated properly, it's able to transport things to your organs they need much more efficiently. Things such as oxygen (you know, that thing we die without?!) as well as the chemical messages, nutrients and hormones they need. Those vital things won't make it where they need to go properly without enough water in your body. When our organs get what they need, they are then able to work properly and we are so much healthier as a result.

Most people don't drink enough water and a lot of the time it's simply because they don't know how much they should be drinking. A few factors need to be taken into account such as your body weight, how active you are, and whether you live in a warm climate or not.

So, first thing first, ascertain how much water you should be drinking. You can do this by taking your weight in kg and dividing it by 0.024. The resultant number is how many millilitres of water you should be drinking every day. You also need to increase your water intake by 350ml for every 30 minutes of exercise.

If you're struggling to get your daily water intake requirement, there are some things you can try. Firstly, if drinking water gets boring for you, try adding things like lemon, cucumber, apple or whatever else you like to make it more interesting. Google can be your best friend if you want to find different variations to try.

Other beverages that DO count towards your daily water intake are teas that don't have caffeine in them and fruit juices. Anything with caffeine in it, such as coffee, soft drinks or normal tea strips water out of your body, so they DO NOT count toward your water intake and should be kept to a minimum.

If you're struggling to get your water intake in because you just plain forget to drink the liquid gold, there are apps you can download to help you remember. Alternatively, you could set an alarm on your phone to go off every 30 minutes to remind you to drink.

I fill up the number of bottles I need to drink each day and know that by the time I go to bed that night, they all have to be finished, which makes it so much easier for me. My body loves me for it and yours will too!

REDUCE PROCESSED FOODS AS MUCH AS POSSIBLE

When I first started writing this chapter, I didn't even think of mentioning this. Not because it isn't important, but because I thought it went without saying. But it occurred to me that while most of us do actually KNOW we should do this, we don't always truly GET it until someone spells it out for us.

So why should we reduce processed foods?

Firstly, anything that has been processed has to have chemicals added to it to keep it from going bad. A lot of those chemicals are just not good for us. It's as simple as that.

Secondly, to make things taste good, all kinds of colours and flavours are added and quite often a lot of sugar or artificial sweeteners. Especially when manufacturers are trying to make something 'low fat'. It tastes like crap when they take the fat out, so they add either a whole heap of sugar or artificial sweeteners.

We all know too much sugar is not good for us, but you would be amazed at how much sugar is in processed foods. Even ones you wouldn't think would be loaded with sugar are. For instance, did you know that there can be the equivalent of up to *four teaspoons* of sugar in ½ a cup of bottled pasta sauce? Or in just two tablespoons of BBQ Sauce? Fruit juices can have up to nine teaspoons of sugar in ONE glass!

Now, I'm not suggesting you totally cut out every single processed food for the rest of your life. If you want to and don't absolutely hate your life that way, go right ahead. But if you're like me, you still want the occasional treat. Hence why I say REDUCE your processed food intake as much as possible.

Finding our healthy doesn't have to be perfect, especially if it means you don't make any changes. Imperfect change is better than none at all!

EAT FRUITS AND VEGETABLES

Most of us don't get anywhere near the servings of fruits and vegetables we should every day. If we want to be healthy, some fruit and lots of vegetables are a must, especially the green, leafy kind. The recommended daily intake is two servings of fruit and five servings of vegetables.

A national survey done in Australia in 2014/2015 showed that 50-55% of men and women were not getting the recommended serving of fruit per day while a staggering 90-95% were not getting their recommended serving of vegetables! For once, this is something that can be ADDED to your nutrition plan, not taken out, so it seems like a no-brainer to me!

Why do we need to eat two servings of fruit and five servings (MINIMUM) of vegetables per day? Because research shows that the more fruit and vegetables we eat, the lower our risk for chronic diseases such as stroke, cancer, type 2 diabetes and heart disease, that's why! So get as many of those beautiful, colourful, vibrant, healing fruits and vegetables in your belly as you can!

GREEN SMOOTHIES!

To help get those extra veggies in that we need, I have a green smoothie almost every day. The thought of a green smoothie might make you gag. I totally get it! I was like that at first too. I promised a friend I would try it though and found – to my surprise – that it actually tasted pretty good! The recipe I was given has fruit in it as well as the green stuff, so although it looks gross (it really does!), it actually tastes yum!

It's an easy way to get a whole lot of extra veggies in one hit, so I highly recommend you give it a try. The recipe for the green smoothie I have every day is on the next page and you'll find many more by using the awesome Google!

The really amazing thing is even if you struggle with it in the beginning, the more of the healthy stuff you get into your body, the more your body will start to crave it. I guarantee that one day, you won't be able to imagine your life without your green smoothie being a major part of it!

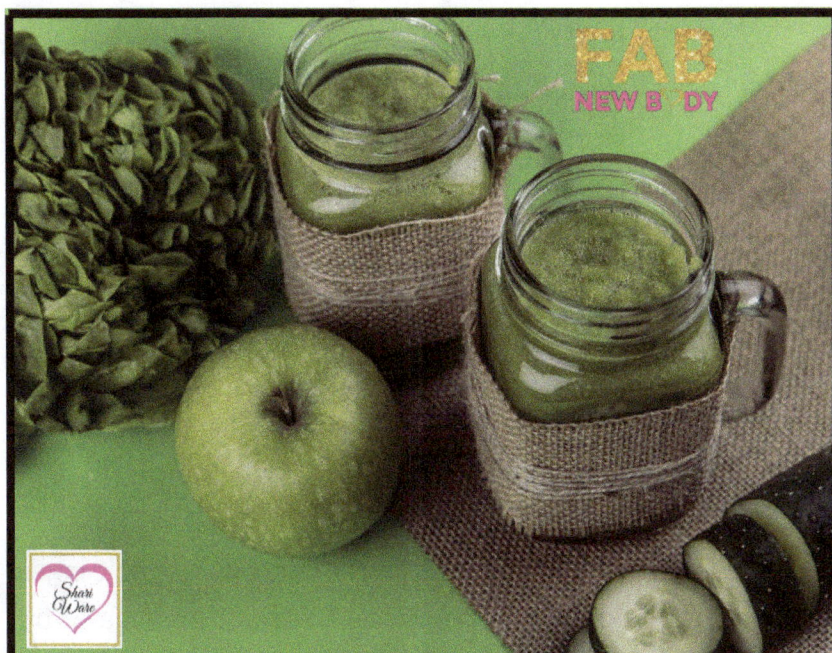

MY GREEN SMOOTHIE RECIPE

30G BABY SPINACH
1/2 LEBANESE CUCUMBER
1 SPRIG OF PARSLEY
10 MINT LEAVES
1/2 LEMON
1/2 APPLE
1CM CUBE GINGER
1CM CUBE TUMERIC
BLACK PEPPER
2 TSP SUPER GREENS
1/2 BEETROOT
150ML WATER

SWITCH TO ORGANIC AS MUCH AS POSSIBLE

Remember the saying, *"You are what you eat"*? We know it's true and that we should eat healthy food as much as possible. The problem these days is that so-called 'healthy' food is not as healthy as we think it is.

For instance, how do farmers keep their crops safe from bugs and pests? They spray them with pesticides, insecticides and herbicides. These chemicals *kill* living animals. We then eat the produce with these chemicals on them. No, we are not as small as the pests they kill, but that doesn't mean we can't ingest enough over a lifetime to cause some serious damage to our bodies. Why take the risk when you can readily source produce that hasn't been sprayed with chemicals and pesticides?

Switching to organic is not only healthier for you, but healthier for the planet, so it's a win-win as far as I'm concerned. You don't need to switch everything at once. Just choose one thing to switch and once you have, don't go back. Then choose the next thing and so on. I'm still in the process of switching to organic and will be for a while, but every time I switch a product to organic, I feel that little bit healthier!

REDUCE SUGAR AND STARCHY CARBS

We know that too much sugar is not good for our body and overconsumption leads to a whole host of problems such as type 2 diabetes, heart disease and obesity. Reducing it as much as possible is definitely going to make you much healthier, especially if you consume a lot.

What a lot of people don't realise is that when they eat starchy carbohydrates such as bread, pasta and rice, they are essentially eating a bucket load of sugar. When these foods are consumed, the body turns them to sugar for energy, so reducing them as much as possible is in the best interest of a healthy body.

Once again, it doesn't mean you have to cut out everything you love entirely. Just work on reducing how much you eat over time.

MAKE HEALTHY SWAPS

If there is something you absolutely love and you know you probably indulge in a little too much, try and find a way to make a healthy swap. For instance, I absolutely love chocolate and refuse to give it up, but I still want to be as healthy as I can. So while I have normal chocolate for an extra special treat from time to time, I have 85% organic dark chocolate most of the time.

Dark chocolate has awesome things like polyphenols and healthy fats which are good for our brain, so I can totally justify having a little bit more often than I would indulge in normal chocolate.

Other healthy swaps could be:

- Organic stevia for sugar
- Zucchini spirals for pasta
- Using wraps instead of bread
- Making your own salad dressings with olive oil and lemon juice.

There are so many healthy swaps you can make so you don't feel as if you are depriving yourself of everything you love.

SLEEP & STRESS

I have put sleep and stress together because they are intertwined. Stress can lead to health problems and one of the biggest stresses that many people have these days is lack of sleep. We are so busy and we try to cram so much into our days that we short ourselves on sleep to find the extra hours in our day. This places major stress on our body and if we have other stresses as well, eventually our health will suffer.

Chronic stress has a major impact on our health. It can lead to fatigue, headaches, high blood pressure, anxiety, obesity, heart disease and diabetes. I explained some of the things that happen to our bodies when we are under stress in Chapter 2 on emotional eating, so go back and check that out if you need a reminder. Long story short though – we need to learn how to turn off the 'fight or flight' switch.

There are several ways you can flip that switch. Firstly, make sure you get a MINIMUM of 6 hours of sleep per night. At least 7.5 hours would be ideal, but if you currently get less than 6, then getting a minimum of 6 as a standard is still going to be a step in the right direction.

Some other ways to turn the switch to the off position are:

- Meditation
- Massage
- Yoga
- Exercise
- Taking time out to socialise with friends and family

EXERCISE

If you don't currently exercise regularly, this is one of the best things you can do for yourself. There are so many benefits of exercise including the fact that it builds and maintains strong muscles and bones, it helps your brain health and memory, it makes you feel happier (endorphins people, endorphins!!), it controls weight, it prevents chronic disease and it promotes better sleep.

Now, I want to be particularly clear that I am talking about MODERATE exercise. Moderate exercise means 150 minutes per week of a moderate activity of your choice – walking, swimming, aerobic exercise and weight bearing activities.

We need to be aware that exercise is also a stress on the body. A certain amount of stress is actually good for us, but as with everything, there is a line. If we take our exercise to the extreme, we are placing too much stress on the body which becomes unhealthy. Exhausting yourself with exercise will do more harm than good in your efforts to create a healthier body.

When I first started exercising, I started with a minimum of three 30-minute sessions per week which contained a mixture of cardio and strength exercises. Both are important for a healthy body. I started out slow and worked my way up to being able to do more over time. Now I usually exercise five to six times per week for 45 minutes per session.

If you struggle to exercise, start by setting yourself a goal that you know you can definitely achieve without too much effort, such as three ten-minute walks per week. When you achieve that goal, you will have scored a win and be motivated to set your new goal a bit higher. Take it slowly and congratulate yourself every step of the way. You are AMAZING!

EDUCATION

I may have put education as number ten on the list, but it's definitely one of the most important ones. We don't know what we don't know. Sometimes we think we're making the healthiest choice for ourselves but unknowingly we're not. This I know from experience and my next book will be about this very subject. But that's the next chapter in the story...

For now, just believe me when I tell you that one of the best things you can do for your health is to commit to learning as much as you can in whatever way you can. Reading books, listening to podcasts, attending health events, etc.

One of the best ways I continue to educate myself daily is by listening to podcasts. I cannot recommend them enough and the knowledge I have gained from them has been life changing and invaluable.

My absolute favourite health and fitness podcast is The Model Health Show with Shawn Stevenson which you can check out at https://themodelhealthshow.com/podcasts/ Another podcast I listen to regularly to help me with motivation, inspiration and self-development is the Tony Robbins podcast which you can find at https://www.tonyrobbins.com/podcasts/. I spend a lot of time in the car and by the time I get to my destination I have a wealth of new knowledge and feel pumped and ready for the next part of my day!

FIND YOUR HEALTHY ACTION STEP

1. Choose two healthier choices from this chapter that you can implement and write them below:

_____

_____

2. Choose one and plan out how you will implement it:

_____

_____

3. Start implementing!

Many small changes add up to MASSIVE change in the end!

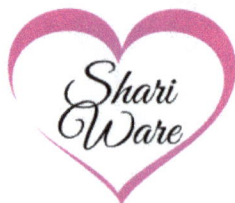

Shari Ware

Chapter Seven

YOU ARE IMPORTANT

This may be the last and shortest chapter of the book, but it is certainly not the least important. In fact, this chapter is one of the MOST important. It's all about YOU and how important YOU are and it's why you will choose some of the healthy choices from this book and *implement* them into your life.

Life today is so busy! There is so much to do and so many of us put everybody else before ourselves. We do for our children, we do for our spouse, we do for our family and friends, but we don't do for ourselves.

When you're on an airplane and they do the safety demonstration, what do they tell you about fitting the oxygen mask if you have children? They tell you to fit your own first and THEN fit your child's. They tell you to do that because you can't help anyone else if you don't take care of yourself first.

YOU are JUST as important as anyone else in your world. You are just as important as your children, you are just as important as your spouse, you are just as important as your family and friends. It's not selfish to take time out to do for YOU. In fact, if you want to be the BEST parent, spouse, family member or friend, then you absolutely need to take the time out to do for you. The more you take care of you, the more you will be able to help others.

These are some of the things I take time out to do for myself every day:

- I practice my self-love rituals

- I practice gratitude

- I meditate

- I draw three angel cards for myself

- I practice my success rituals

- I indulge my secret guilty pleasure of Pokémon Go for at least 15 minutes every day!

Find some things you love to do and take time out for yourself to do them. It doesn't have to be complicated or cost money. If you love reading, it can be as simple as taking time out to read one chapter of a book. It could be taking a bath. It could be a massage. As long as it feeds your soul in some way, it totally counts!

YOU are IMPORTANT! Yes... YOU!

FIND YOUR HEALTHY ACTION STEP

1. Write down two things you know you don't do for yourself but would like to:

    _____

    _____

2. For each of the two things, write down how it will positively affect your life if you implement them:

    _____

    _____

3. Choose one and implement it today!

4. Watch my video at https://youtu.be/T3wuc8IIIaE for some final tips to help you on your journey to finding YOUR healthy!

YOU

are

important

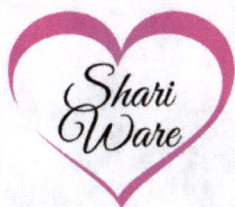

About the Author

AUTHOR BIO

Weight Loss Mindset Mentor and #1 Best Selling Author Shari Ware went from slicing a piece of cake, to slicing her weight in half! In fact, she spent more than a decade in the morbidly obese classification and was fortunate that no major health crisis came her way.

Shari now helps others win the weight battle the way she did – one change at a time. Shari has made it her mission to help others change their story and find their HEALTHY. She discovered the secret to successfully releasing weight and found that it applies to every goal that we set for ourselves in life. Now she helps others to find their WHY Power as a critical starting point which, in conjunction with making a series of changes over a period of time, leads to massive change.

Other tools that Shari has added to her toolbelt to help people are a Personal Training qualification and a certification in Hypnotherapy, NLP and Life Coaching. She's been featured by That's Life Magazine, Take 5 and New Idea as well as appearing on Today Tonight, the Channel 9 Morning Show and Channel 9 News. Shari has also been featured in various Australian and UK online news publications such as The Telegraph and The Courier Mail.

If you would like to connect with Shari and find out how she helps people to overcome Mephobia and change their story in various ways, including helpful and practical tips, you can do so on Facebook at https://www.facebook.com/shariwarefab/

I hope you enjoyed this book! Please feel free to share it with friends and post a review so I can help more people to find THEIR healthy!

Shari Ware
Weight Loss Mindset Mentor
xoxo

DON'T FORGET TO:

Book a complimentary 30-minute call with me to find your healthy!

https://calendly.com/shari-ware/30min

Connect with me on Facebook – Shari Ware

https://www.facebook.com/shariwarefab

Connect with me on Facebook – FAB New Body

https://www.facebook.com/fabnewbody

Connect with me on Instagram

https://www.instagram.com/shariwarefab

Connect with me on Twitter

https://twitter.com/shariwarefab

Connect with me on Linked In

https://www.linkedin.com/in/shariware

#1 Best Selling Author of Fat to Fabulous – Diet Free Weight Loss for Real Women

You can get the book here: https://amzn.to/2E0sqSl

Imperfect change is better than NO change. Just make a change!

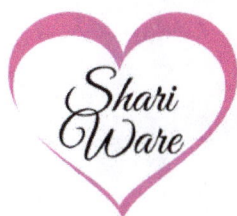

Shari Ware